Navigating the Change: A Woman's Guide to a Healthy Menopause Transition

Navigating the Change: A Woman's Guide to a Healthy Menopause Transition

Table of Content

Introduction: Your Menopause Roadmap

Menopause is a natural transition that all women experience as they age. It marks the end of your reproductive years and ushers in a new phase of life. While a significant milestone, menopause is often shrouded in misconceptions, fears and uncertainties. Many women lack the information and support needed to make this change as smooth and positive as possible.

This book provides the roadmap to understand and thrive during the menopausal transition. It aims to empower you with practical solutions for common symptoms, along with lifestyle tips to optimize your wellbeing. You'll learn to view menopause not as an ending, but as an opportunity to reinvent and transform yourself.

Understanding Your Transition

The lead-up to menopause, known as perimenopause, starts for most women in their mid-40s. It is characterized by fluctuating ovarian function and estrogen levels. This hormonal rollercoaster can last anywhere from 2 to 8 years.

The physical symptoms arise from these hormonal shifts. You may experience hot flashes, night sweats, vaginal dryness, sleep disturbances, weight gain, and slowed metabolism. Psychological symptoms can include irritability, anxiety, depression, mood swings, memory lapses, and reduced motivation. You may also notice changes in your sexuality and relationships.

While symptoms differ for each woman, it helps to know what to expect so you can be proactive. Monitoring your cycle and hormone levels equips you to manage this transition. Lifestyle measures like proper sleep, nutrition, exercise and stress relief can provide relief without necessarily needing medications. Complementary wellness practices also support this adjustment.

Reframing Perspectives

Menopause has historically been portrayed negatively - as a milestone marking the end of youth and fertility. But modern women are redefining this outlook. Instead of just surviving menopause, the goal is to thrive by blossoming into your wisest, most empowered and authentically expressed self.

The key is to reframe your perspective by seeing menopause as a beginning, not an ending. It ushers in new possibilities for personal growth, healthy aging, and living life on your own terms. This time of change can strengthen your self-confidence, sense of freedom, and commitment to self-care.

Your Wellness Toolbox

This book equips you with an array of tools to navigate menopause transitions gracefully. You'll learn practical strategies to manage symptoms, balance hormones, and optimize energy and mood. Lifestyle changes to boost heart health, strengthen bones, improve sleep quality, and maintain a healthy weight are covered.

Holistic remedies, stress management techniques, emotional health practices, sexual wellness, and strengthening relationships are also addressed. Most importantly, you'll gain insights to embrace this next chapter of your life with optimism, power, and joy.

Consider this book your guide and companion during the menopause journey. Use it to understand the changes happening in your body, as well as to nurture your emotional, mental and spiritual well-being. With knowledge, self-care and healthy lifestyle choices, you can move through menopause feeling empowered and discovering new vitality.

The navigation has begun - let's explore the course together!

Part I: Understanding Menopause

Before you can successfully navigate menopause, it's helpful to start with a strong understanding of what it really entails. This first part of the book will explore:

- What happens in your body during perimenopause and menopause

- The short-term and long-term physical changes

- The common symptoms you may experience

- The impact on your emotional health and mood

- How your sexuality and relationships may change

Having accurate information about what to expect will help you be proactive in managing this transition.

Perimenopause is the 2 to 8 year transitional phase leading up to menopause. It's characterized by fluctuating hormones, disrupted cycles, and the start of symptoms. Menopause officially begins 12 months after your last menstrual period, marking the end of fertility.

The key change is the decline in ovarian estrogen production. Estrogen regulates many functions in the body, so this drop causes widespread effects. Lower estrogen levels impact everything from your menstrual cycles to body temperature regulation, metabolism, heart health, bone density, bladder function, lubrication, and more.

Understanding the physiology will help you understand why you may experience hot flashes, night sweats, vaginal dryness, mood swings, sleep disturbances, and other common symptoms. Education is empowering, so you can make informed choices about lifestyle changes, holistic options, and medical treatments.

While menopause ends your fertility, it is not the end of your femininity or sexuality. With care and communication, you can ease discomfort and maintain intimacy in relationships. Practicing self-compassion will help you through mood swings and challenging days.

Navigating the biological, emotional, sexual and psychological facets of this change is much smoother when you understand what's happening. Let's explore each one so you can develop a toolbox of solutions. Knowledge is power – knowing what to expect will help you manage the changes gracefully and gracefully.

Onward to understanding!

Chapter 1: What is Menopause?

Menopause is a natural biological process that all women experience as they age. It marks the end of your reproductive years and your menstrual cycles. The transition into menopause is a gradual one, occurring over several years. This time of hormonal shifts produces both physical and emotional changes.

Let's start by getting clear on the terminology and stages of the menopausal transition.

Stages of Menopause

There are three overall stages:

Perimenopause

Perimenopause means "around menopause" and refers to the 2-8 year transitional phase leading up to the final menstrual period. It typically begins in your 40s, but can start earlier or later.

During perimenopause, estrogen levels fluctuate and ovulation becomes irregular. You may notice cycle changes like longer or shorter periods, lighter or heavier flow, or cycles spaced closer together or further apart.

The hormonal ups and downs often produce menopausal symptoms like hot flashes, night sweats, vaginal dryness, irregular bleeding, trouble sleeping, and mood changes. However, you are still considered premenopausal during this stage.

Menopause

Menopause is reached after you've gone 12 consecutive months without a menstrual period. At this stage, the ovaries have stopped releasing eggs and estrogen/progesterone production decreases significantly.

The average age for menopause is 51, but it can occur anywhere from 40-55. Premature menopause before age 40 affects about 1% of women.

The common symptoms of perimenopause may continue or worsen in early menopause. Long-term effects like bone loss and increased heart disease risk also begin.

Postmenopause

This refers to the stage after menopause has occurred, starting when 12 months have passed since your last period.

Hormone levels stabilize at their new lower levels during postmenopause. Vasomotor symptoms like hot flashes ease for most women, but other physical changes persist in the absence of estrogen.

Long-term health risks are a greater concern now and continue until the end of life. Maintaining good nutrition, activity levels, and preventative care is important in postmenopause.

What Causes Menopause?

Menopause occurs due to the natural depletion of ovarian follicles - the sacs that contain immature egg cells. At birth, women have about 1-2 million follicles. This number drops over time, with only about 1000 remaining by puberty.

Each month, follicles mature and release an egg for potential fertilization and pregnancy. By age 50, most of the follicles are gone and egg production declines. With low estrogen output from the ovaries, menstrual cycles become irregular and eventually stop.

Natural menopause is a consequence of ovarian aging. The follicles essentially "run out" at an average age of 51. But certain medical conditions can trigger premature menopause earlier than normal:

- Premature ovarian failure - follicles stop functioning before 40

- Surgical removal of the ovaries for medical reasons

- Cancer treatments like radiation or chemotherapy

- Autoimmune disorders

Menopause should not be confused with an intentional cessation of fertility, like with tubal ligation. It is due to the ovaries' decreased capacity for hormone and egg production.

Effects of Low Estrogen

Estrogen helps regulate many processes in the female body. So the hormone depletion has widespread effects:

- Irregular menstrual cycles and cessation of fertility

- Vasomotor instability - hot flashes and night sweats

- Vaginal/urogenital atrophy - dryness, thinning, irritation

- Sexual dysfunction - low libido, painful intercourse

- Bladder issues - urinary urgency/frequency

- Accelerated bone loss, higher fracture risk

- Adverse changes in cholesterol, higher cardiac risk

- Loss of collagen, skin/tissue changes

- Sleep disturbances, fatigue, memory lapses

- Joint pain or stiffness

- Emotional fluctuations - depression, anxiety, irritability

These changes are most pronounced in the 1-5 years after menopause. Effects like bone loss and heart disease risk persist long-term. Managing symptoms and staying healthy after menopause involves balancing risks and hormones.

Key Takeaways

- Menopause is the point when menstruation ceases due to ovarian aging and lowered estrogen levels. It signals the end of fertility.

- Perimenopause is the 2-8 year transition period leading up to menopause, with irregular cycles and fluctuating hormones.

- Symptoms arise from the estrogen decline and can persist for years after menopause.Long-term health risks also increase after menopause.

- Understanding what to expect will empower you to make healthy choices to manage this transition smoothly.

Now that you understand the basics of menopause, let's explore the perimenopausal transition and its effects. Knowledge is power!

Chapter 2: Perimenopause - The Lead-Up

Perimenopause marks the beginning of your body's transition into menopause. During this stage, your reproductive system starts shifting toward changes that will ultimately culminate in menopause. Let's look at what happens during this phase.

What Happens During Perimenopause

As outlined in chapter 1, perimenopause refers to the transitional stage before menopause when hormone levels begin to fluctuate. It typically spans 2-8 years.

Several key changes occur:

- Estrogen levels start to rise and fall unevenly, often sharply dropping
- Menstrual cycles become irregular - longer, shorter, lighter, or heavier
- Ovulation happens inconsistently and fertility declines
- The intervals between cycles may be shorter or longer
- Changes in cervical mucus and vaginal tissue
- Emergence of menopausal symptoms like hot flashes

You are still considered premenopausal during this phase, as ovulation is still occurring even if sporadically. Perimenopausal hormone changes are a consequence of ovarian aging. The follicles that produce eggs and hormones start deteriorating.

Blood levels of the follicle stimulating hormone (FSH) begin to rise as the ovaries respond less to stimulation. FSH prompts the ovaries to grow and release eggs. As ovarian function wanes, FSH increases to compensate.

So in perimenopause you have aging ovaries producing fewer eggs and less estrogen coupled with rising FSH as the body tries to kick them into action. These changes set the stage for full-blown menopause.

Recognizing the Start of Perimenopause

Most women realize perimenopause has begun due to recognizable cycle changes:

- Menstrual periods become irregular and unpredictable

- Unusually long (35+ days) or short (less than 21 days) cycles

- Heavier, lighter or shorter periods

- Spotting between periods

- Skipped or missed periods

Symptoms like hot flashes, night sweats, sleep troubles, mood changes, and vaginal dryness often start in perimenopause as well. There may be breast pain or tenderness too.

Some also experience heart palpitations, dizziness, headaches, electric sensations in the legs, and gastrointestinal issues as part of hormonal fluctuations.

Ovulation prediction kits can track ovulation patterns. Tracking BBT curves can reveal cycle irregularity too. FSH blood tests help, as levels over 25-30 mIU/ml may indicate perimenopause.

The unpredictability of perimenopause can be frustrating. But anticipating changes will help you respond proactively. Monitoring cycles and symptoms enables you to manage fluctuations better.

Coping With Unpredictable Cycles

To handle irregular periods:

- Carry panty liners or pads, menstrual cups, pain relievers

- Keep extra clothes/underwear in case of accidents

- Use a period tracker app to record flow, mood, symptoms

- Notice patterns - do changes align with certain weeks?

- Discuss sudden heavy bleeding with your doctor

- Try supplements like maca root or vitex to regulate hormones

- Reduce stress and maintain healthy lifestyle

Be prepared for your period to come unexpectedly, change flow levels mid-cycle, or go missing some months. This erraticism is part of the perimenopausal hormone rollercoaster. Discuss very heavy bleeding with your doctor to ensure no fibroids or other issues.

Overall, see this time as an opportunity to get in tune with your body's changes. Tracking and self-care will help smooth the transition into menopause.

Key Takeaways

- Perimenopause starts the hormonal fluctuations leading to menopause, lasting around 2-8 years on average.

- Estrogen levels begin to drop unevenly, FSH rises, and ovulation happens inconsistently.

- Menstrual cycles often become longer, shorter, lighter or heavier and very unpredictable.

- Symptoms like hot flashes, vaginal changes, and sleep disruption often emerge.

- Monitor your cycle patterns and communicate with your doctor during this transition.

- Be prepared for unpredictable periods and implement lifestyle measures to cope.

Stay tuned for Chapter 3, which outlines the many symptoms associated with the decline in estrogen during perimenopause and into menopause. Understanding these effects is key to managing them proactively.

Chapter 3: Physical Changes and Symptoms

The hormone fluctuations leading up to and during menopause trigger a wide range of physical effects. These occur as the body adjusts to declining estrogen levels. Understanding the potential symptoms will help you identify them early and respond appropriately.

In this chapter, we'll outline the short-term symptoms related to hormonal changes as well as long-term health risks that increase after menopause.

Vasomotor Symptoms

Vasomotor symptoms arise from estrogen's role regulating body temperature and vasodilation, the widening of blood vessels. As estrogen drops, the brain's temperature regulation center becomes impaired. This triggers:

Hot Flashes

- Brief sensations of intense warmth and flushing, often with sweating and red skin

- May be accompanied by rapid heartbeat, anxiety, skin tingling, dizziness or weakness

- Typically last 1-5 minutes

- Frequency ranges from occasional to constant

- More common at night and triggered by stress, alcohol, hot drinks

Night Sweats

- Hot flashes occurring at night, often severe enough to wake you or soak the bedding

- Can disrupt sleep quality and cause fatigue, irritability, moodiness

- Gradually improve in frequency and intensity in postmenopause

Not all women get hot flashes or only have mild ones. Genetics, ethnicity, and lifestyle factors play a role. Managing triggers, dressing in layers, and lowering ambient temperatures can provide relief. Some also benefit from prescription or herbal therapies.

Vaginal/Bladder Changes

The vaginal walls have estrogen receptors that stimulate collagen production and maintain thickness, elasticity, and lubrication. After menopause:

- Vaginal tissue becomes thinner, less elastic, more fragile

- Vagina shortens and narrows

- Less vaginal fluid and lubrication is produced, creating dryness

- Increased risk of irritation, inflammation, infections

- Discomfort or pain during intercourse

- More frequent urination or incontinence

- Higher risk of UTIs

These changes develop over 1-5 years as estrogen levels continue to decline. Using lubricant and maintaining vaginal health through regular intercourse or dilator therapy can help prevent atrophy. Some may benefit from prescription estrogen creams or pills to improve tissue quality if symptoms are severe.

Sexual Dysfunction

In addition to the physical changes that can hamper sex, many women experience a lowered libido and sexual responsiveness after menopause due to:

- Hormone changes - estrogen and testosterone both affect desire

- Vaginal discomfort or pain during sex

- Fatigue, sleep disorders, mood changes, stress

- Body image issues after childbearing years

- Interpersonal issues or partner sexual dysfunction

Over-the-counter lubricants, moisturizers, and creams can improve comfort. But counseling, lifestyle changes, and stress management may be needed to address libido or arousal issues not fixed by topical treatments.

Open communication and intimacy building activities can help overcome relationship challenges. Some women also choose bioidentical hormone replacement with testosterone to enhance libido.

Other Physical Effects

Additional impacts from menopause include:

Skin, breast and hair changes: Declining estrogen reduces collagen, causing skin to become thinner and less elastic. Breasts lose volume as fat tissue decreases. Hair may thin.

Weight gain/body fat redistribution: Fat accumulates more around the abdomen versus hips and thighs. Slower metabolism makes weight loss harder.

Heart palpitations: Hormone changes can disrupt the electrical system, causing skipped beats or palpitations. These are usually harmless but check with your doctor.

Headaches: Fluctuating estrogen can trigger migraines or headaches in some women. These often improve after menopause.

Joint pain: Lower estrogen accelerates bone loss and can worsen conditions like osteoarthritis. Joints may ache from normal activity.

Gastrointestinal issues: Digestive upsets like bloating, gas, and IBS can accompany perimenopause. Crashing estrogen levels affect gut motility.

Gum/dental issues: Estrogen loss is linked to gingivitis, gum recession, and tooth loss in some women.

Tingling extremities: Some feel crawling or prickly sensations in their limbs, likely from fluctuating hormones. It's harmless but annoying.

Breast tenderness: Shifting hormones cause breast soreness or tenderness, similar to PMS symptoms, in some women.

Allergies/asthma: Surges and drops in estrogen affect immune response, which can worsen allergies and asthma symptoms. These often improve after menopause.

Brain fog: Trouble concentrating, memory lapses, and cloudy thinking result from hormonal effects on cognition and brain activity.

Staying active, managing stress, eating nutritiously, and getting quality sleep are helpful for minimizing these symptoms during the menopausal transition.

Long-Term Health Risks

In addition to short-term symptoms, lower estrogen after menopause increases risks for certain conditions over time:

Osteoporosis: Accelerated bone loss occurs in the absence of estrogen's bone-protective effects. This raises susceptibility to fractures and breaks.

Cardiovascular disease: Declining estrogen is associated with adverse cholesterol changes that can lead to plaque buildup in arteries. Heart attack and stroke risks increase.

Urinary incontinence: Weakened pelvic floor and urethral muscles make leakage with exercise, coughing, laughing more likely.

Weight gain/obesity: Fat accumulation, especially visceral belly fat, coupled with slowed metabolism, can lead to overweight or obesity.

Diabetes: Postmenopausal women have a higher likelihood of developing type 2 diabetes due to insulin resistance and weight gain.

Cognitive decline: After menopause, women may be more susceptible to dementia-related memory loss and decline in thinking skills.

Certain cancers: Lower estrogen is tied to increased risks of colon, pancreatic, and other system cancers in postmenopausal women.

Through healthy lifestyle choices, you can effectively minimize risks and even gain strength after menopause. We will cover specific wellness strategies in Part II.

Key Takeaways

- Menopause transition symptoms arise from declining and fluctuating estrogen. Effects range from hot flashes to sexual changes.

- Vaginal dryness, discomfort with sex, and incontinence are common after menopause.

- Long-term risks like osteoporosis, heart disease, diabetes, and cancer increase.

- Know what to expect so you can identify symptoms early and implement effective management.

- Maintaining a healthy lifestyle helps counteract risks and minimize disruptive symptoms.

Stay tuned for Chapter 4, which delves into the psychological symptoms and mood changes many women encounter during the menopausal transition.

Chapter 4: The Effects on Mood and Mental Health

In addition to the physical impacts covered in Chapter 3, many women experience changes in mood and mental health during the menopausal transition. The hormonal fluctuations involved can affect emotions and brain function.

Let's explore the common psychological symptoms, their causes, and healthy ways to manage them.

Depression

Depressed mood or clinical depression affects about one in four women transitioning into menopause. Some contributors include:

- Estrogen regulates serotonin, dopamine, and endorphins which affect mood. Unstable levels can disrupt this balance.

- Night sweats and sleep disturbances from lower estrogen impair quality rest needed for emotional equilibrium.

- The realization of aging, children leaving home, career shifts, and other life changes may trigger situational depression.

- Premenstrual dysphoric disorder (PMDD) can worsen with hormonal instability.

Milder depressive symptoms may lift after menopause is complete and hormones stabilize. But clinical depression should be treated through counseling, antidepressants if warranted, and lifestyle changes like exercise, healthy eating, and stress relief.

Support groups, introspection tools like journaling, and activities that bring joy and purpose can also help overcome depressive periods.

Anxiety

Many women experience surges of anxiety during the menopausal transition as well:

- Estrogen calms the brain's worry center, so drops can stimulate anxiety. Adrenaline surges from hot flashes don't help.

- Unpredictable cycles and menopause symptoms can provoke worries over loss of control.

- Sleep disruptions make it harder to cope with stressors.

- Life changes like career shifts, empty nests, illness, or death of loved ones may underlie the anxiety.

- For some, fluctuating estrogen aggravates existing anxiety disorders.

Relaxation techniques, regular exercise, therapy, anti-anxiety medications if needed, meditating, and cognitive behavioral therapy (CBT) can help manage anxiety. Getting social support and making time for enjoyable activities also helps.

Irritability and Mood Swings

Many women report feeling more irritable, sensitive, or emotionally volatile during the menopausal transition. Some contributing factors include:

- Estrogen, serotonin, and other hormones influencing mood rise and fall unevenly.

- Hot flashes and night sweats interrupt sleep, leaving you fatigued and on edge.

- The emotional impact of changing roles, identities, and life circumstances.

- Feeling out of control of your body and emotions.

Strategies like tracking mood swings to identify patterns, exercising to relieve stress, finding social outlets, and fostering self-compassion can help smooth out mood variability. This symptom often gradually resolves as hormones rebalance.

Trouble Concentrating and Memory Lapses

"Brain fog" and impaired cognition are common complaints, attributed to:

- Estrogen supports memory, learning, and focus. Declining levels hamper these cognitive processes.

- Changes in neurotransmitters that facilitate brain function.

- Sleep disruptions and stress/anxiety also undermine concentration.

- For some, normal age-related impairment seems accelerated.

Memory aids, brain-stimulating activities, stress management, exercising, eating brain-boosting foods, and getting quality sleep can help counteract effects on concentration and memory. Staying mentally active and social seems to help too.

Low Motivation and Fatigue

Women commonly report decreased motivation, apathy, lethargy, and fatigue during the menopausal transition as well. Causes include:

- Drops in energizing estrogen leave you feeling drained. Adrenal fatigue from hormonal stress may play a role too.

- Changes in brain chemicals like serotonin, dopamine and endorphins sap motivation.

- Sleep troubles from night sweats and insomnia hamper daily energy.

- Anemia from heavy periods can contribute to exhaustion.

- Thyroid issues may also cause fatigue.

Boosting energy with exercise, restorative yoga, adequate nutrition, iron and vitamin D, thyroid testing, and medication if indicated, addressing sleep issues, and coaching for motivation/life balance can help overcome this symptom.

Key Takeaways

- Menopausal hormonal changes can negatively impact mood, mental health and cognition in some women.

- Depression, anxiety, irritability, memory and concentration issues are common complaints.

- Causes include shifting estrogen, neurotransmitters, sleep issues, life stresses, and loss of control.

- Lifestyle measures, social support, therapy, and medication when needed can help manage symptoms.

- Tracking patterns and triggers will help you find effective coping strategies.

Stay tuned for Chapter 5, which explores the effects of menopause on sexuality and intimate relationships between partners.

Chapter 5: Impact on Sexuality and Relationships

In addition to the individual physical and emotional changes outlined in earlier chapters, the transition into menopause often affects relationships and sexuality for partnered women.

Declining hormone levels combined with vaginal changes can hamper intimacy, arousal, and satisfaction. Relationship dynamics may shift too during this life stage.

Let's explore these sexual and interpersonal effects in more detail:

Physical Intimacy and Sexual Satisfaction

As discussed in Chapter 3, the urogenital changes that accompany menopause - including vaginal dryness, thinning tissues, irritation, and pain - can interfere with intercourse, arousal, orgasm and pleasure. Lower estrogen also reduces libido and responsiveness for many women.

additional factors like fatigue from poor sleep, body image issues, medications, other menopausal symptoms, and pre-existing sexual dysfunctions also contribute to sexual issues.

Strategies like using vaginal lubricants and moisturizers, maintaining intimacy through touching and oral sex when intercourse is uncomfortable, slow sexual play, and integrating sex toys like vibrators help overcome physical obstacles.

But sexual changes often have an emotional impact too, which we'll cover later in this chapter.

Partnership Support

How intimate partners respond to and support women coping with menopausal changes also influences relationship satisfaction. Those who display understanding, encouragement and patience report greater happiness.

Whereas partners who shame, criticize or isolate themselves from menopausal women increase distress. Teasing about things like memory lapses or weight gain erodes self-esteem. Mocking hot flashes or night sweats shows a lack of empathy.

Good communication about symptoms, intimacy needs, and how partners can thoughtfully help makes the transition easier on relationships. Counseling helps when partners need guidance communicating constructively.

Changing Roles and Identities

For some couples, the shifts in roles and identities that coincide with midlife and empty nests negatively impact relationship dynamics and satisfaction.

As women's reproductive roles end and they evolve professionally, socially, or through new creative outlets, relationships may destabilize if partners don't support their growth and identity changes.

Counseling helps partners mourn losses mindfully while embracing new directions. Introspective work like journaling, support groups, and couples activities fosters self-discovery and resets bonds on more empowering dynamics.

Sexual Self-Perception

Body image often suffers during the menopausal transition as weight gain redistributes fat, skin loses elasticity, and breasts change. Seeing oneself as less sexually attractive can hamper libido and arousal.

Affirming inner dialogues, mindfulness practices, exercising for health versus weight loss, and focusing more on body sensations versus appearances improves sexual confidence.

Finding non-appearance based compliments and expanding definitions of sensuality also help counteract the emphasis on conventional attractiveness.

Emotional Impact of Sexual Changes

Even with supportive partners, women often report negative emotions like frustration, anger, inadequacy or embarrassment over symptoms affecting their sexuality, like vaginal pain.

Letting go of rigid expectations about sex, prioritizing sensual touch and emotional intimacy, redefining sex beyond intercourse, and sharing vulnerabilities with partners helps relieve shame.

Professional counseling, support groups, and self-compassion practices enable women to gain perspective and work through the complex feelings related to sexual changes.

Key Takeaways

- Physical menopausal changes combined with shifting roles affects relationships.

- Good communication and partner support eases this transition.

- Women may need to adjust self-perceptions and sexual expectations.

- Counseling and mindfulness help relieve complex emotions about sexual function.

- Maintaining intimacy through creative touch, playfulness and emotional bonding is important.

That concludes Part I covering the key things to understand about the menopausal transition. Next we'll explore strategies and healthy behaviors to help smooth symptoms and risks during this change. Knowledge is power!

Part II: Strategies for Wellbeing

Now that you understand what happens during perimenopause and menopause, it's time to equip you with strategies to navigate this transition with grace and ease.

While menopause brings unavoidable changes, how smoothly you experience this shift depends largely on your lifestyle and self-care choices. The right habits and behaviors can significantly relieve bothersome symptoms and optimize wellbeing.

This second part of the book provides practical solutions in key areas:

- Managing hot flashes, night sweats and improving sleep
- Easing vaginal discomfort and maintaining healthy intimate relations
- Keeping your heart strong, bones resilient and weight steady
- Balancing hormones and finding natural symptom relief
- Fueling your body with the right nutrition to minimize risks
- Incorporating movement, activity and mindfulness for optimal wellness
- Understanding when medications may be helpful

Armed with this toolbox of tips and techniques, you'll be able to respond to menopausal changes proactively and effectively. Small tweaks can yield big improvements in your quality of life.

While menopause brings changes beyond your control, your behaviors and lifestyle are well within your control. Focus on the aspects of health and wellbeing you can optimize.

With the right knowledge, you can thrive and flourish during the menopausal transition and beyond. Perimenopause and menopause are opportunities for self-care, growth and nurturing new life phases.

Turn the page as we dive into healthy habits and healing solutions to help you look and feel your best!

Chapter 6: Managing Hot Flashes and Night Sweats

Hot flashes and night sweats are some of the most commonly reported menopausal symptoms. These sudden sensations of intense warmth with flushing and sweating can range from mildly annoying to severely disruptive for women.

Fortunately, many effective remedies and lifestyle changes can provide relief by preventing, reducing or managing hot flashes.

In this chapter, we'll outline both medical and natural solutions to ease vasomotor symptoms.

Understanding Hot Flashes

As outlined in Chapter 3, hot flashes result from decreasing estrogen levels, which impair the body's ability to regulate temperatures. This causes sudden dilating of blood vessels and flushing.

When the brain's thermostat malfunctions, it reads the body's temperature as too high, triggering sweating and rapid heat loss responses. After a few minutes, the hot flash subsides.

Hot flash triggers include:

- Stress, anxiety or strong emotions

- Warm environments and weather

- Caffeine, spicy foods, alcohol

- Tight clothing and layers that obstruct heat loss

- Smoking and tobacco use

Tracking your personal triggers and patterns helps you avoid or better manage hot flashes. Vaginal estrogen can relieve symptoms for some women. But lifestyle measures and other natural remedies may provide adequate relief.

Medical Therapies

If hot flashes are severe and interfere with work, sleep and quality of life, medical therapies include:

Hormone therapy (HT) - Estrogen alone or with progestin alleviates hot flashes in most women. Oral tablets, skin patches, gels, sprays and vaginal rings deliver relief. However, HT has risks like blood clots, stroke and breast cancer that limit its use.

Antidepressants - Low doses of certain SSRI and SNRI drugs ease hot flashes, likely by regulating brain serotonin and temperature centers. Venlafaxine and desvenlafaxine show efficacy. Side effects include sexual dysfunction.

Gabapentin - This anti-seizure drug reduces hot flash severity by regulating brain pathways involved in temperature. Side effects include dizziness and fatigue.

Clonidine - This blood pressure medication may decrease hot flash frequency and intensity for some women by lowering the "set point" temperature that triggers flushing.

Discuss benefits and risks of these therapies with your healthcare provider. Often lifestyle measures can provide adequate relief without medication risks.

Lifestyle Changes and Natural Remedies

Making certain lifestyle adjustments and using evidence-based natural remedies can significantly decrease hot flash frequency and intensity:

Dress in breathable, layered clothing - Light, loose layers that can be shed allow sweat evaporation and cooling. Natural breathable fabrics help too.

Lower ambient temperatures - Cooler room temperatures prevent overheating episodes. Use fans, open windows and set AC to around 68-72°F.

Practice deep breathing - At the onset of a hot flash, take long slow breaths to promote relaxation and heat dissipation. Deep belly breathing triggers the rest/digest response.

Keep hydrated - Drinking at least 64 ounces of cool water daily helps regulate body temperature. Being well-hydrated prevents overheating.

Manage triggers - Identify and avoid personal hot flash triggers like caffeine, alcohol, spicy foods, stress and warm environments.

Exercise regularly - Physical activity, even moderate walking, improves thermoregulation and lowers the severity of hot flashes.

Practice relaxation techniques - Yoga, meditation, massage and guided imagery relax the nervous system and may lessen hot flashes. Managing stress helps.

Try botanical remedies - Supplements like black cohosh, soy isoflavones, and red clover may decrease hot flashes due to their estrogenic plant compounds, per some studies.

Get sufficient sleep - Restorative sleep enhances the body's ability to regulate temperature. Prioritize good sleep hygiene.

Eat phytoestrogen foods - Soy, flaxseeds, sesame seeds, oats, and legumes contain natural plant estrogens that may temper hot flashes.

Consider cognitive behavioral therapy (CBT) - CBT focused on menopause teaches coping strategies that can reduce hot flash intensity.

Avoid smoking and limit alcohol - Smoking and drinking exacerbate hot flashes. Quitting smoking and reducing alcohol helps.

With some diligent lifestyle adjustments and evidence-based natural remedies, bothersome vasomotor symptoms can be managed effectively in many women.

Key Takeaways

- Hot flashes result from decreased estrogen and impaired temperature regulation.

- Hormone therapy is very effective but confers health risks that limit usage.

- Non-hormonal medications like SSRIs, gabapentin or clonidine may help.

- Simple lifestyle measures like dressing in layers, lowering room temperature, and avoiding triggers provides substantial relief for many women.

- Natural remedies, mindfulness practices, CBT and healthy habits also decrease hot flash frequency and severity.

In the next chapter, we'll cover solutions for night sweats and improving sleep quality, which commonly disturb rest during menopause.

Chapter 7: Easing Vaginal Dryness and Discomfort

As estrogen levels fall during perimenopause and menopause, declining amounts of this hormone reach receptors in the vaginal tissue. This causes significant changes.

The vaginal walls grow thinner, less elastic, and more fragile. Lubricating mucous production decreases, creating dryness. Low estrogen also disturbs the pH balance and healthy bacteria in the vagina.

This atrophic vaginitis, or vaginal atrophy, can cause irritation, burning, itching, painful urination, bleeding with sex, increased infections, and discomfort during intercourse.

Let's explore the options available to relieve vaginal dryness and related discomforts. Both over-the-counter remedies and prescription treatments provide relief.

Over-the-Counter Moisturizers and Lubricants

Using vaginal moisturizers and lubricants is often the first line of treatment for mild to moderate vaginal dryness and associated pain or itching. These provide temporary relief and comfort.

Moisturizers hydrate vaginal tissues and mimic lost mucous secretions. Used regularly, they relieve irritation and supplement the vagina's natural lubrication. Replens and K-Y Liquibeads are common brands.

Lubricants coat the vaginal walls and vulva to reduce friction during intercourse. Water- or silicone-based lubricants like Astroglide, K-Y Jelly, and Pjur are safe with condoms. Oil-based types may damage latex.

Apply moisturizers daily as needed for ongoing relief. Use lubricants as needed before and during sexual activity. Continued use helps prevent thinning of vaginal tissues.

Prescription Estrogen Therapy

For moderate to severe vaginal atrophy symptoms, prescription estrogen preparations help rejuvenate delicate tissues and restore thickness and elasticity. They may also reduce recurrent urinary tract infections.

Vaginal estrogen creams - Low-dose estradiol or conjugated equine estrogen creams, rings or tablets are inserted directly into the vaginal canal using an applicator. They deliver concentrated hormones to vaginal tissue with less systemic effects.

Oral estrogen pills - Low doses of estrogen tablets like Premarin provide systemic relief. But higher circulating estrogen increases risks like blood clots, so vaginal routes are preferred.

Discuss the benefits and risks of each method thoroughly with your healthcare provider. Localized, low-dose therapies are considered safe for most women with moderate to severe vaginal atrophy.

Using prescription estrogen vaginally also does not interfere with the efficacy of hormone-positive breast cancer treatments like aromatase inhibitors.

Staying Sexually Active

Continuing to have intercourse regularly - or inserting dilators if penetration is too uncomfortable - helps maintain elasticity and thickening of the vaginal walls.

Physical stimulation increases blood flow and promotes healthier tissue. If intercourse is painful, engage in sexual play to keep tissues primed. Vaginal health deteriorates further without regular dilation and stimulation.

Alternative Therapies

Phytoestrogen botanicals like soy, red clover, black cohosh, and dong quai consumed orally or applied vaginally may provide mild estrogenic effects to improve vaginal lubrication and elasticity. Data is limited, but some women report relief.

Vitamin E - Applying vitamin E oil to the vulva and entrance of the vagina acts as a natural lubricant and moisturizer. It should not be inserted deeply.

Vitamin D - Correcting any vitamin D deficiency may help improve vaginal cell growth and repair. Vitamin D also has anti-inflammatory effects.

ThermiVa - This gentle radiofrequency laser treatment stimulates new collagen and elastin to help tighten and rejuvenate vaginal tissue. It requires multiple sessions and has minimal side effects.

Key Takeaways

- Declining estrogen causes vaginal and vulvar dryness, thinning, irritation, and pain. This worsens after menopause.

- Non-hormonal moisturizers and lubricants provide immediate relief for mild symptoms.

- Low-dose vaginal estrogen reverses more severe atrophy and discomfort in most women.

- Staying sexually active keeps tissues more elastic. Self-dilation with dilators also helps if sex is too painful.

- Alternative remedies may offer mild relief in some cases but lack strong clinical evidence.

- Addressing vaginal discomfort can help maintain intimacy and sexual satisfaction.

Next we'll discuss strategies for improving sleep quality, which is often significantly disrupted during the menopausal transition.

Chapter 8: Coping with Sleep Disruptions

Up to 60% of women report sleep disturbances during perimenopause and menopause. Sleep becomes lighter, more fragmented, and prone to disruption. This results in fatigue, impaired concentration and moodiness.

Hot flashes and night sweats frequently interrupt sleep. But hormonal fluctuations also impair sleep quality independent of vasomotor symptoms. Fortunately, both medical treatments and healthy sleep habits can restore restorative slumber.

Let's review why menopausal sleep suffers and solutions to overcome insomnia and other issues.

Causes of Menopausal Sleep Disorders

Several factors contribute to disrupted sleep patterns:

- **Nocturnal hot flashes and sweating** - These nighttime vasomotor symptoms directly interrupt sleep continuity.躰突drenching the bedding.

- **Anxiety and mood changes** - Fluctuating estrogen and progesterone heighten anxiety and depression in some women, impairing ability to fall and stay asleep.

- **Hormone effects on sleep circuits** - Estrogen modulates GABA receptors, serotonin, melatonin and other neurotransmitters involved in regulating sleep-wake cycles. Declining levels impair these cycles.

- **Poor sleep hygiene** - Behaviors like inconsistent bedtimes, electronic use before bed, and unstable routines hamper quality sleep.

- **Other medical issues** - Sleep apnea, restless legs, and chronic pain conditions also erode sleep.

- **Medications** - Some drugs like steroids, stimulants and certain antidepressants disturb sleep architecture.

Evaluating all potential contributors through sleep studies and other medical tests allows appropriate treatment. Simple lifestyle measures also help significantly.

Medical Treatment Options

If self-care strategies don't resolve moderate to severe menopausal insomnia or night sweats, medical therapies include:

- **Hormone therapy** - Systemic estrogen or progestin therapy prevents hot flashes that disrupt sleep. Local vaginal estrogen may help too. However, hormones haverisks that limit long-term use.

- **Antidepressants** - Selective serotonin reuptake inhibitors (SSRIs) like fluoxetine relieve hot flashes and may promote deeper sleep.

- **Gabapentin** - This nerve pain medication reduces night sweats and improves sleep quality in some women.

- **Clonidine** - This blood pressure drug diminishes night sweats and hot flashes for some by stabilizing body temperature regulation.

- **Sleep aids** - Short-term use of medications like zolpidem, eszopiclone and Belsomra treat insomnia, but may lose effectiveness over time and confer side effects.

Discuss all medication options thoroughly with your physician to make personalized choices based on your health profile and sleep study results. Lifestyle measures should be tried first.

Lifestyle and Home Remedies

Numerous behavioral strategies and natural remedies improve sleep quality during menopause before medications are necessary:

- **Keep a consistent sleep schedule** - Maintain the same bedtime and wake-up time, including weekends. This stabilizes the circadian clock.

- **Optimize sleep hygiene** - Make your bedroom cool, dark and quiet. Don't use phones/TVs before bed. Avoid stimulating activities.

- **Reduce hot flash triggers** - Avoid spicy foods, caffeine, alcohol and stress for 4 hours before bedtime.

- **Lower ambient temperature** - Cooler ambient temperatures prevent night sweats that disrupt sleep.

- **Try cognitive behavioral therapy (CBT)** - CBT targets thought patterns and behaviors impairing sleep. It's as effective as medications.

- **Take melatonin** - This sleep-regulating hormone supplement helps initiate drowsiness. Time-released versions improve efficacy.

- **Have a pre-bed routine** - Activities like chamomile tea, stretching, journaling and hypnosis recordings ready your mind for quality rest.

- **Exercise daily** - Regular physical activity, especially morning workouts, promote deeper REM sleep. Avoid vigorous exercise before bed.

- **Manage stress and anxiety** - Relaxation practices like yoga, meditation, and mindfulness calm your mind from daily stresses that impair sleep.

Adjusting environment, habits and thought patterns can resolve menopausal insomnia for many women without medications. Seek medical advice if self-care strategies and sleep hygiene don't help after a month.

Key Takeaways

- Hot flashes and hormone changes often disturb sleep quality during menopause.

- Medical therapies like hormones, antidepressants and sedatives can treat moderate/severe sleep disorders.

- But healthy sleep habits, relaxation practices and CBT improve sleep for most women without drugs.

- Maintain consistent bedtime routines and wind-down rituals to promote restorative sleep.

- Address anxiety, hot flash triggers and sleep environment for better nighttime comfort.

Stay tuned for Chapter 9, which details other strategies, habits and lifestyle changes to balance energy and fight fatigue during menopause. Sleep and activity work hand in hand for optimal wellbeing.

Chapter 9: Maintaining Energy Levels and Fighting Fatigue

Fatigue and depleted energy levels afflict up to 45% of perimenopausal and menopausal women. Hormone fluctuations, poor sleep, stress, anemia, thyroid issues and simple aging all conspire to sap vitality.

Building habits and routines that renew energy allows you to combat exhaustion and restore motivation. Let's examine why menopause saps energy and key ways to promote resilient stamina.

Causes of Menopausal Fatigue

Several factors cause menopausal and perimenopausal fatigue:

- **Poor sleep** - Insomnia and night sweats from hormonal shifts impair sleep quantity and quality. Lack of deep REM sleep leaves you drained.

- **Iron deficiency anemia** - Heavy menstrual bleeding depletes iron reserves needed to produce energizing red blood cells.

- **Thyroid issues** - These develop in some women as metabolism slows, provoking fatigue.

- **Blood sugar swings** - Dropping estrogen alters glucose metabolism and may lead to hypoglycemic dips in energy.

- **Adrenal changes** - Constant stress may trigger adrenal fatigue, leaving you depleted.

- **Cardiovascular effects** - Lower estrogen facilitates small vessel changes that reduce oxygen circulation.

- **Nutrient deficiencies** - Menopause increases needs for iron, magnesium, B vitamins and vitamin D to produce energy.

- **Lifestyle habits** - Sedentary routines, poor diet, chronic stress and lack of coping skills magnify exhaustion.

- **Mood disorders** - Depression and anxiety drain motivation and initiative.

Evaluating all contributing factors allows you to implement the appropriate solutions to restore vibrant energy as you navigate menopause.

Medical Management of Fatigue

If self-care measures don't relieve disabling exhaustion, consult your doctor to assess possible medical causes and treatments:

- **Thyroid medication** - Levothyroxine can correct hypothyroidism. Thyroid levels should be evaluated.

- **Iron supplements** - Iron tablets or intravenous iron corrects deficiency anemia to improve blood oxygen carrying capacity.

- **Antidepressants** - If depression or anxiety underlie fatigue, medications often help resolve low motivation and apathy.

- **Blood sugar medication** - Metformin or other drugs can stabilize blood glucose variations that lead to energy crashes.

- **Adrenal support** - Adaptogenic herbs, hydrocortisone, or DHEA may boost adrenal function in severe fatigue, under medical supervision.

- **Hormone therapy** - Estrogen or combined therapy can lift fatigue, but long-term use has significant risks.

Lifestyle measures alone help many, but don't hesitate to seek medical advice if exhaustion persists despite self-care.

Lifestyle Strategies to Boost Energy

Numerous lifestyle habits and behaviors build resilience and renew energy levels naturally during menopause:

- **Exercise regularly** - Aerobic activity, strength training and yoga boost endorphins, improve oxygenation and build vitality. Even light activity helps.

- **Eat frequent small meals** - Eating protein, complex carbs and healthy fats every 3-4 hours maintains blood sugar and energy balance.

- **Reduce sugar and refined carbs** - These lead to reactive hypoglycemia and energy/mood crashes. Limit intake.

- **Stay hydrated** - Being well-hydrated is essential for energy production. Aim for 64 ounces of water daily.

- **Take a multivitamin** - A high-quality multivitamin covers any nutrient gaps dragging down energy.

- **Treat sleep disorders** - Using sleep hygiene strategies, cognitive behavioral therapy, and physical activity restores restorative rest to help fatigue.

- **Practice relaxation techniques** - Yoga, meditation, massage, and deep breathing activate the rest/digest nervous system to recharge you.

- **Engage in hobbies** - Pursuing enjoyable hobbies and creative pastimes provides uplifting mental distraction to boost motivation.

- **Increase plant foods** - Fruits, vegetables and whole grains provide sustained energy and help stabilize blood sugar.

Don't tolerate fatigue as inevitable. Numerous lifestyle remedies and natural therapies can restore vibrant energy to carry you through menopause and beyond.

Key Takeaways

- Fatigue and lack of motivation are common menopausal complaints.

- Contributing factors range from poor sleep to thyroid issues, blood sugar instability and mood disorders.

- Medical assessment determines if thyroid drugs, iron, antidepressants or other treatments are warranted.

- But healthy habits like better nutrition, activity, sleep hygiene, stress management and hobby pursuit can often lift low energy without medications.

- Don't settle for exhaustion. Implement lifestyle strategies to restore resilient stamina.

In the next chapter, we'll detail nutrition and diet approaches to keep your heart strong, bones resilient, and weight steady during the changes of menopause.

Chapter 10: Keeping Your Heart and Bones Strong, Weight Steady

The drop in estrogen during menopause accelerates aging-related changes like bone loss and cardiovascular decline. But diet and lifestyle adjustments can counteract these risks to keep your heart strong, bones resilient and weight steady.

Optimizing nutrition provides key building blocks to support your body through hormonal changes. Let's review eating strategies to minimize menopause risks.

Bone Health

Estrogen helps maintain healthy bone density by facilitating calcium absorption and bone growth. Postmenopausal estrogen decline is tied to accelerated bone loss. This increases susceptibility to osteopenia, osteoporosis and fractures.

Dietary approaches to keep bones strong include:

Get enough calcium - Adults need 1000-1200 mg of calcium daily. Dairy products, leafy greens, beans, salmon, and fortified foods provide calcium. Supplement if diet is inadequate.

Include magnesium - Magnesium optimizes calcium absorption and bone mineralization. Good sources include spinach, avocado, nuts, seeds, beans and whole grains.

Increase vitamin D - Vitamin D aids calcium absorption and bone building. Get 400-800 IU/day through sunshine, fortified dairy/juices and fatty fish. Supplement if deficient.

Eat fruits and vegetables- Produce provides bone-supporting nutrients like potassium, vitamin K, and antioxidants. Shoot for 5-9 servings per day.

Choose animal proteins - Meat, poultry, fish, eggs and dairy provide protein to build and preserve lean muscle and bone mass. Aim for 0.5 grams of protein per pound of body weight daily.

Reduce salt- High sodium intake interferes with calcium retention, so keep sodium intake under 2300 mg per day.

Limit caffeine - High caffeine intake interferes with calcium absorption, so keep coffee and tea intake moderate.

Minimize bone-depleting foods - Limit excessive protein, sugary sodas, alcohol and processed foods high in phosphorous which impair bone density.

Quit smoking - Smoking reduces estrogen and weakens bones. Quitting reverses bone loss.

Weight-bearing and resistance exercise are also essential to build and maintain bone strength. Walking, strength training, yoga and Tai Chi benefit bones.

Heart Health

Declining estrogen is associated with rises in LDL cholesterol, lower HDL, increased plaque buildup, and higher risk of cardiovascular disease after menopause.

Diet strategies to protect your heart include:

Eat phytoestrogen foods - Soy, flax, oats and legumes contain plant estrogens that may balance cholesterol.

Choose healthy fats - Omega-3 fatty acids in salmon, avocados, olive oil, nuts and seeds support heart health. Limit saturated fats.

Increase fiber - Soluble fiber in oats, nuts, beans, apples, and carrots helps lower LDL cholesterol.

Eat antioxidant-rich foods - Fruits, vegetables and green tea provide antioxidants that prevent cholesterol oxidation and plaque formation.

Use herbs - Garlic, ginger, turmeric, cinnamon and rosemary have natural anti-inflammatory effects that benefit circulation and arteries.

Drink alcohol moderately - If you drink, limit alcohol to 1 drink daily. Too much raises blood pressure and heart disease risks.

Quit smoking - Smoking damages arteries and significantly elevates risks for heart disease, stroke, and heart attack in all women.

Reduce sodium - Limiting sodium prevents fluid retention and improves heart failure risk factors.

Manage stress - Chronic stress contributes to cardiovascular risks. Relaxation practices like yoga lower stress hormones.

Exercise aerobically - Aerobic activity keeps your heart strong, circulation robust, and prevents plaque buildup in vessels.

Following heart-healthy dietary patterns such as the Mediterranean diet provides a nutritious approach to keep your cardiovascular system strong after menopause.

Maintaining Healthy Weight

Weight gain and altered body composition are common complaints during the menopausal transition. Shifting hormones and aging both impact metabolism, body fat storage, and weight management.

Strategies to maintain healthy weight include:

Eat plenty of produce - Fruits and non-starchy vegetables provide nutrients and fiber for fewer calories. They optimize digestion and keep you fuller longer.

Choose whole grains - Minimally processed whole grains like brown rice, quinoa, and oats stabilize blood sugar and make you feel satiated. Limit refined grains.

Include plant protein - Beans, lentils, nuts, seeds and soy offer filling plant-based protein and fiber without excess saturated fat.

Eat fish - Fatty fish provides anti-inflammatory omega-3 fats that improve body composition.

Hydrate well - Drinking adequate water prevents false hunger signals caused by mild dehydration. Filtered water is best.

Spice it up - Spices like cayenne, turmeric, cinnamon and ginger boost metabolism slightly.

Limit portion sizes - Being mindful not to overeat, especially high-calorie processed foods and desserts, prevents weight gain.

Exercise regularly - Aerobic and resistance exercise helps maintain lean muscle mass and revs metabolism. Even walking benefits metabolic rate.

Get 7-9 hours of sleep - Poor sleep disruption cues hunger hormones that stimulate appetite and fat storage.

Balancing nutrition, activity and other lifestyle factors allows you to maintain a healthy weight and feel your best during menopause.

Key Takeaways

- Bone loss, heart disease risks and weight gain intensify during menopause.

- Optimizing calcium, vitamin D, antioxidants, fiber and healthy fats helps protect bone and heart health.

- Lean proteins, produce, whole grains, and spices support healthy weight management.

- Regular exercise provides important benefits for bones, heart and metabolism too.

- Support your body through hormone changes with nourishing diet and active lifestyle habits.

In the next chapter, we'll explore the pros and cons of commonly used supplements and natural remedies for managing menopausal symptoms.

Chapter 11: Natural Remedies and Lifestyle Changes for Symptoms

Many women look to natural and complementary options to manage menopausal symptoms like hot flashes, sleep issues, and vaginal dryness without medications. Certain lifestyle remedies, herbs, vitamins, and supplements may help provide relief.

Let's examine the evidence for popular natural therapies for menopausal discomforts. Work with your doctor to evaluate safety and effectiveness for your profile.

Hot Flash Therapies

Phytoestrogens - Soy foods, flax, red clover and other sources of plant estrogens may have mild effects on hot flashes due to their estrogen-mimicking compounds. Data is mixed. Use food sources instead of concentrated supplements.

Black Cohosh - Several studies find this herb effective for reducing hot flash frequency and severity. It has a good safety profile at recommended doses. May provide estrogen-like activity.

Evening primrose oil - Primrose and other sources of gamma-linolenic acid (GLA) show modest benefits for hot flash reduction in some studies. Safe to try.

Vitamin E - Some clinical evidence supports vitamin E supplements (400-800 IU/day) to relieve hot flashes, especially in breast cancer survivors. Safe at moderate doses.

Acupuncture - Regular acupuncture treatments reduce hot flash frequency and intensity for many women. It likely activates temperature regulation pathways. Minimal side effects with licensed acupuncturists.

Cognitive behavioral therapy (CBT) - CBT focused on menopause teaches techniques to reduce stress responses and perceive hot flashes as less bothersome. Some positive studies.

Stellate ganglion block - This anesthetic nerve block procedure temporarily reduces hot flash intensity, but benefits only last up to 3 months. Used as a diagnostic tool.

Herbal products have the most robust support but confer mild side effects in some women, like stomach upset. Lifestyle remedies like acupuncture and CBT may also help relieve vasomotor symptoms.

Sleep and Fatigue Aids

Melatonin - This sleep-regulating hormone in supplement form helps initiate drowsiness. May improve sleep quality, but not duration. Short-term use is considered safe.

Valerian - Some evidence indicates valerian root capsules shorten the time to fall asleep and improve sleep quality. Generally safe but can cause headaches.

Magnesium - Magnesium aids sleep and muscle relaxation. Try 150-300mg before bed, in forms like glycinate or citrate. Also helpful for nighttime leg cramps.

Adaptogens - Herbs like ashwagandha, rhodiola and maca help counteract stress and balance hormones related to fatigue. Reasonably safe, but can be stimulating.

CoQ10 - This antioxidant energizes cellular energy metabolism. Some women note reduced fatigue when taking 100-200mg daily. Few side effects.

Ginseng - Siberian and Asian ginseng have traditionally been used to fight fatigue and boost vitality. Limited clinical evidence, but quite safe. May be stimulating.

B vitamins - A B-complex supplement or multivitamin ensures you get enough B vitamins for converting food into energy. Deficiencies can cause tiredness.

Iron - Have ferritin levels checked as iron deficiency is a common cause of menopausal fatigue. Supplement if indicated and monitor labs. Constipation is a side effect.

Herbs, melatonin, and magnesium have the strongest evidence for aiding sleep. Vitamins play a supporting role in energy metabolism. Work with your healthcare provider before supplementing.

Mood Enhancers

St. John's Wort - This herbal extract is well-studied for reducing mild to moderate depression and anxiety. However, it interacts with many medications. Use cautiously under medical guidance.

Sam-E - This supplement stands for s-adenosyl methionine and may help relieve depressive symptoms. Avoid if you have bipolar disorder.

5-HTP - Derived from tryptophan, 5-HTP may increase serotonin to improve mood balance. Do not combine with antidepressants.

Saffron - This spice contains antioxidants shown in clinical studies to be as effective as antidepressants for milder depression. Generally safe.

Omega-3 fatty acids - Fish oil and other sources of anti-inflammatory omega-3s may help regulate mood. Include oily fish in your diet or take up to 2 grams of supplements.

Vitamin D - Correcting any vitamin D deficiencies may improve depression. Get levels tested before supplementing with 2000-5000 IU per day.

Exercise - Aerobic exercise and yoga have strong evidence for stress relief and mood-lifting effects. Aim for 30 minutes daily. Safe and free!

Herbs like saffron and St. John's Wort have promising effects but may not be right for everyone. Discuss supplement and medication interactions with your doctor.

Key Takeaways

- Herbal remedies, vitamins and natural therapies may help manage disruptive menopausal symptoms.

- Phytoestrogens, black cohosh, and cognitive therapy show efficacy for hot flashes. Melatonin and magnesium aid sleep.

- For low mood, omega-3s, saffron, Sam-E and exercise have demonstrated effects in studies.

- Discuss medication interactions and get lab testing to ensure safety and efficacy if using supplements.

- Use remedies as complementary options along with healthy lifestyle habits for optimal wellbeing.

Next we'll provide more extensive guidelines for developing habits and behaviors focused on self-care, nutrition, activity and mindfulness to smooth your menopause transition.

Chapter 12: Incorporating Movement, Mindfulness and Self-Care

While hormone changes are outside your control, you have full control over lifestyle habits that profoundly affect menopausal symptoms. Experts now consider healthy behaviors the foundation for wellbeing during this transition.

In this chapter, we'll provide guidelines for exercise, activity, mindfulness practices, and holistic self-care to help you feel vibrant and flourish through perimenopause and beyond.

Exercise and Activity

Being physically active provides multiple benefits for common menopausal symptoms:

- **Improves hot flashes** - Regular activity regulates body temperature, improves thermoregulation, and decreases hot flash frequency and intensity for most women. Even lighter exercise helps.

- **Eases mood changes** - Aerobic exercise boosts serotonin, endorphins and endorphin production to balance mood and relieve anxiety and depression.

- **Stabilizes energy** - Movement energizes by improving circulation, triggering the release of stimulating neurochemicals, and combating fatigue.

- **Promotes better sleep** - Daily exercise helps consolidate sleep cycles, increasing deeper REM and total sleep time for many women.

- **Maintains heart health** - Active women have lower risks for cardiovascular disease after menopause by keeping blood vessels flexible and heart strong.

- **Strengthens bones** - Weight bearing activities like walking, dancing, jogging and strength training stress bones in a positive way to retain density and reduce osteoporosis risk.

- **Manages weight** - Exercise helps counteract the drop in resting metabolism that often occurs during menopause. Activity helps regulate appetite hormones too.

Aim for 150 minutes per week of moderate exercise like brisk walking or cycling, plus two strength sessions to retain muscle mass. Yoga provides additional benefits. But any movement helps!

Mind-Body Practices

Techniques that elicit the "relaxation response" balance the stress hormones exacerbating menopausal symptoms like hot flashes, insomnia, and mood instability. Beneficial mind-body practices include:

Yoga - Research confirms yoga reduces anxiety, depression, and vasomotor symptoms significantly. Gentle styles increase comfort.

Meditation - Meditating practices focused on controlled breathing, mantras or awareness calm brain circuits involved in body temperature, sleep, mood and stress response. Apps like Calm provide guided meditations.

Hypnosis - Hypnosis and guided imagery programs designed for menopause help control hot flashes and improve sleep quality based on clinical trials.

Tai Chi - This gentle martial art elicits relaxation while building balance and strength. It may reduce menopausal insomnia and stress as well as yoga and meditation.

Breathwork - Diaphragmatic belly breathing triggers relaxation pathways. Try 4-7-8 breathing - inhale for 4 seconds, hold for 7, exhale for 8.

Acupuncture - Regular treatments reduce hot flashes and depression in women transitioning through menopause. You can try weekly.

Mindfulness - Practices and cognitive therapy that increase present moment awareness, self-compassion and resilience modulate stress and discomfort.

Restorative Self-Care

Nurturing mind, body and spirit bolsters coping skills to manage menopause changes gracefully. Consider adding:

- **Healthy nutrition** - Choose whole, nutrient-dense foods to nourish yourself well during hormone shifts. Stay hydrated.

- **Massage** - Weekly massage lowers cortisol, alleviates anxiety, and improves sleep. Trade with a partner or try chairs at the mall.

- **Nature time** - Spending time outdoors lifting your mood. Forest bathing, gardening, and green exercise reduce stress.

- **Therapy** - Talk therapy provides support and helps develop coping strategies. Join group counseling focused on midlife transitions.

- **Community** - Sharing experiences with friends,virtual communities or support groups builds solidarity. You're not alone!

- **Spiritual practices** - Activities providing meaning and purpose such as volunteering, creativity, or religious community involvement enhances wellbeing.

- **Self-care rituals** - Treat yourself to relaxing baths, soothing music, uplifting books, or other practices that replenish your spirit.

Key Takeaways

- Daily movement, mind-body techniques, nourishing foods, community and therapeutic self-care habits all profoundly influence menopause experience.

- Regular exercise provides the most significant benefits for common symptoms from hot flashes and depression to sleep, weight and energy.

- Yoga, meditation, massage, nature and calming practices counteract stress and discomforts.

- Building happiness through fulfilling activities and relationships nourishes resilience.

- Make self-care priority number one during this transition!

In the final chapter, we'll provide a roadmap for developing personalized approaches by identifying your top priorities and most bothersome symptoms.

Part III: Emotional Wellness

While the physical changes of menopause have received more attention historically, supporting emotional health is equally important for wellbeing as estrogen levels shift.

Perimenopause and menopause can be challenging transitions—the ending of fertility, changing roles, aging, and symptoms all affect mood and outlook. A holistic approach addresses mindset and emotions along with the physical.

In Part III, we'll explore strategies to:

- Smooth out emotional ups and downs

- Reduce anxiety and depressive symptoms

- Manage stress skillfully

- Cultivate self-compassion and resilience

- Rediscover meaning and purpose

- Strengthen intimate relationships

- Reignite your sexuality and sensuality

- Embrace this stage of life with optimism

Emotional health habits like therapy, mindfulness practices, intimacy building, creative outlets, and community support groups help women navigate midlife changes with insight and grace.

While some sadness, grief or distress over aging, shifting roles, and lost fertility are normal, you can move through the transition to emerge wiser and more empowered.

Let's delve into practices for mastering your mental health, nurturing relationships, appreciating your evolving identity, and infusing this stage of life with happiness. With the right tools, this passage can be enriching, liberating and even joyful!

Chapter 13: Navigating Emotional Changes

Many women experience emotional ups and downs as hormones fluctuate leading up to menopause. Sudden mood swings, irritability, anxiety, sadness and depression are common complaints.

Understanding what causes these emotional changes and learning coping strategies allows you to smooth out rough patches and maintain an even keel. Let's examine healthy ways to balance your mood.

Causes of Menopausal Mood Changes

As outlined in earlier chapters, declining and unstable estrogen levels disrupt neurotransmitters and hormones that influence emotions and mood, like serotonin, endorphins, and cortisol.

Specifically, dropping estrogen levels can:

- Decrease serotonin, leading to anxiety or depression

- Trigger norepinephrine surges, causing irritability

- Disrupt cortisol rhythms, affecting stress response

- Reduce endorphins that boost mood

In addition to hormonal effects, stress, poor sleep quality, low energy, and life changes during this transitional time can challenge emotional equilibrium.

Recognizing that unstable moods arise from fluctuating hormones and life stresses helps you respond compassionately rather than self-critically when you feel off kilter.

Healthy Ways to Regulate Mood

When hormones are in flux, the key is to implement healthy self-care habits that create emotional anchors and stability during the menopause transition:

Exercise regularly - Aerobic exercise, yoga, and strength training boost mood-regulating neurotransmitters and endorphins while lowering stress hormones. Moving daily lifts mood.

Practice meditation - Meditation and breathwork elicit the relaxation response to calm the mind and nervous system. Try apps like Calm for guided meditations.

Do creative activities - Pursuing creative outlets and hobbies you enjoy elevates mood by releasing feel-good brain chemicals associated with flow states.

Spend time in nature - Being outdoors and connecting with nature has clinically proven mood-boosting effects by reducing cortisol, anxiety, and negative thoughts.

Getenough sleep - Prioritize 7-9 hours nightly, maintain sleep hygiene habits, and treat disorders contributing to fatigue, which exacerbates emotional fragility.

Eat nourishing foods - A balanced diet rich in plants, anti-inflammatory fats, and gut-healthy fiber stabilizes energy and mood by balancing blood sugar and neurotransmitters.

Take a long view - Remind yourself fluctuating moods are temporary and will improve as hormones rebalance in the postmenopausal phase.

Lean on community - Turn to social support, friends, family, counseling groups, or virtual communities to feel connected through changes.

Practice self-care - Do little daily acts that replenish you mentally, physically and spiritually, like enjoying calming music, decluttering or treating yourself.

Try therapy - Talk therapy is extremely effective for working through menopause or midlife stresses that affect your mood and outlook.

Be patient and compassionate with yourself on days when your mood feels off. Implementing healthy, uplifting habits will help smooth out emotional fluctuations.

Managing Anxiety

Many women experience increased anxiety as perimenopause begins, which can worsen from poor sleep, low energy, hot flashes and life stresses. Hormone changes directly affect anxiety by:

- Decreasing calming serotonin

- Increasing stimulating norepinephrine

- Disrupting cortisol and stress regulation

In addition to everyday anxiety symptoms like excessive worry, muscle tension, pounding heart rate or sweaty palms, some women experience anxiety attacks or bursts of severe anxiety with heart palpitations, dizziness or shortness of breath.

The same healthy habits that balance mood - exercise, meditation, community, therapy - also reduce anxiety by lowering stress hormones and activating relaxation pathways.

Additional anxiety-taming tips:

- **Limit stimulating substances** - Caffeine, alcohol, and added sugars can exacerbate anxiety by provoking swings in blood sugar or adrenaline.

- **Try CBD oil** - CBD has a calming effect without the psychoactive effects of marijuana. Follow dosage on quality products.

- **Use grounding techniques** - Tactile or sensory experiences like holding a textured stone, smelling essential oils, or listening to soothing music brings you into the present moment and interrupts the anxious mind.

- **Challenge anxious thinking** - Counseling helps reframe worrying thoughts and limiting beliefs fueling anxiety into more realistic perspectives.

Do progressive muscle relaxation- This involves tensing and relaxing muscle groups to release physical tension that feeds anxiety. Apps provide guided relaxations.

Anxiety often arises from feeling out of control. Using healthy habits, community support, and self-care rituals will help create an anchor of stability.

Overcoming Depression

Up to 1 in 4 women experience depression during the menopausal transition. Causes include:

- Estrogen effects on neurotransmitters like serotonin, dopamine and endorphins

- Fatigue from poor sleep

- Stress from changing roles and life events

- Grief and sense of loss over aging or children leaving home

Sadness, crying spells, low motivation, changes in appetite, and feeling emotionally flat or hopeless are symptoms.

In addition to the mood-lifting habits outlined above, remedies include:

Take antidepressants if warranted - Your doctor may prescribe SSRI or SNRI medications to correct neurotransmitter imbalances contributing to depressive symptoms. These are very effective for many.

Correct hormone imbalances - Lab testing for thyroid, iron, vitamin D, estradiol and testosterone levels helps determine if deficiencies are exacerbating low mood. Replace as needed.

Counteract negative thinking - Cognitive behavioral therapy (CBT) teaches skills to challenge pessimistic thoughts and beliefs that influence depression. This rewires mental habits.

Go to counseling - Working with a therapist provides crucial support, helps you process emotions, and equips you with coping strategies. Consider joining a depression support group too.

Treat sleep apnea -Undetected sleep apnea worsens fatigue and mood issues. Get tested for this common disorder that increases in midlife women. Using a CPAP machine helps.

Use light therapy - Daily exposure to bright light, especially early morning, helps regulate melatonin, cortisol and other hormones tied to seasonal or menopausal depression. Try light boxes.

Depression should never be accepted as "normal", even though it is common. Seeking solutions through counseling, medications as needed, and healthy lifestyle habits alleviates symptoms so you can enjoy life fully again.

Key Takeaways

- Menopause hormone changes commonly trigger mood swings, anxiety, irritability and depression.

- Regular exercise, calming practices, community and therapy help smooth variable emotions.

- For anxiety, limit stimulants, use grounding and muscle relaxation techniques, and challenge worried thinking.

- Seek counseling and consider antidepressants if moderate to severe depression develops. Also correct any hormone imbalances.

- With the right tools, you can ride out temporary mood changes and emerge emotionally stronger than ever!

Chapter 14: Stress Management and Self-Care

Coping with stress effectively is especially vital during the menopausal transition. Stress exacerbates common symptoms and speeds aging if not skillfully managed.

Building self-care rituals, relaxing your nervous system through various practices, and organizing your life reduces the daily stress burden. Let's explore techniques to master stress.

Impacts of Stress

Your body is designed to mount temporary "fight or flight" responses to perceived dangers through surging stress hormones like cortisol and adrenaline. But chronic activation of this response over long periods damages health.

Stress worsens menopausal symptoms by:

- Increasing cortisol, which interferes with estrogen balance

- Depleting serotonin and other relaxing brain chemicals

- Magnifying emotional reactivity, anxiety and depression

- Disrupting sleep cycles, leading to fatigue

- Impairing immune response and triggering inflammation

- Promoting abdominal weight gain

Learning stress reduction techniques offsets these amplified symptoms and risks during menopause. Stress management should be priority number one.

Relaxation Practices

Activities that trigger the relaxation response reverse the deficits of excess stress, lowering heart rate, respiration, blood pressure and muscle tension. Benefits start immediately. Try:

- **Deep breathing** - Inhale deeply, drawing breath into the belly. Exhale slowly. Repeat for 5 minutes whenever stressed.

- **Progressive muscle relaxation** - Systematically tense and relax muscle groups throughout the body to release tension. Apps provide guidance.

- **Guided imagery** - Use relaxing visualized scenes, affirmations or hypnosis recordings to enter a calm, focused state. Imagery activates brain areas that quiet stress circuits.

- **Yoga and meditation** - These practices elicit profound relaxation and balance hormone systems regulating stress reactivity. Even 5 minutes helps.

- **Tai chi, qigong and massage** - Gentle movement and massage techniques decompress the body and mind. Schedule regular massages.

- **Time in nature** - Being in natural settings lowers cortisol, blood pressure and heart rate within minutes. Try forest bathing, gardening or outdoor exercise.

Expressive arts - Crafting, drawing, dancing or playing music engages your senses, provides creative outlet and shifts focus away from stressful thoughts.

Practice relaxation techniques daily, especially when feeling stressed or before bedtime. They provide fast-acting relief without side effects.

Organize and Simplify

Ongoing life stresses pile onto menopausal changes. Getting organized helps reduce feeling frantic and overwhelmed:

- **Use planners and calendars** - Record all obligations to visualize time commitments. Schedule priorities first before filler tasks.

- **Block distracting websites/apps** - Limit time spent compulsively checking low-value sites that steal time and focus.

- **Keep a running to-do list** - Downloading all obligations onto a list frees up working memory, providing a sense of control. Prioritize urgent tasks and chip away steadily.

- **Delegate if possible** - Enlist help from family, hire professionals, or use prepared meal services to ease burdens.

- **Tackle clutter** - Physical clutter creates subconscious stress. Take 15 minutes daily to organize, sort and purge piles.

- **Set boundaries** - Limit work hours, be judicious about volunteering, and learn to say no to nonessential requests. Funnel energy to what matters most.

Practice mindfulness - Stress often arises from dwelling on the past or worrying about the future. Mindfulness meditation trains focus on the present moment. Apps like Headspace teach techniques.

Organization systems, simplifying obligations, and controlling technology use prevents stress buildup. Keep life's demands in check.

Key Takeaways

- Stress exacerbates menopausal symptoms by stimulating cortisol and fight-or-flight pathways.

- Relaxation practices like deep breathing, yoga, nature exposure and massage counteract stress.

- Organizing schedules, decluttering, setting boundaries and practicing mindfulness also reduces stress.

- Make stress relief a top priority through restorative self-care activities and efficient organization.

- Mastering stress improves your ability to smoothly navigate menopausal changes and minimize disruptive symptoms.

In the next chapter, we'll explore practices that build resilience, positivity and healthy perspectives to master your mental health during menopause.

Chapter 15: Cultivating Resilience and Positivity

Adopting habits and perspectives focused on resilience, personal growth, gratitude and positivity will help you navigate the menopause transition with grace and ease.

Learning to accentuate the positive sets the stage for this new phase of life to be enriching and meaningful. Let's explore practices to cultivate an uplifting mindset.

Resilience - Bouncing Back from Challenges

Resilience is the ability to cope with hardship or change in a flexible, optimistic way so you can bounce back and even grow stronger. Building resilience helps you handle menopause's ups and downs skillfully. Ways to boost resilience include:

Foster optimism - Focus on positive aspects, express gratitude regularly, use affirmations, and visualize goals met. Train your brain to filter for the positive versus ruminating on the negative.

Connect with community - Building strong social ties and support networks creates emotional anchors during challenging times. Share your experience with others.

Learn and grow - Stretch yourself to gain new skills. Enjoy classes, workshops and intellectual challenges. Learning boosts self-confidence.

Practice self-care - Nurturing yourself physically, mentally and spiritually makes you more emotionally resilient. Do little daily acts just for you.

Look for meaning - When faced with difficulties, ask how you can learn from the situation or help others. Finding purpose promotes post-traumatic growth.

Celebrate small wins - Recognize any progress made, not just big goals reached. Small gains build positivity momentum.

Use calming practices - Meditation, yoga, deep breathing, and time in nature regulate your stress response so everyday hassles feel less overwhelming.

Keep perspective - When you feel frustrated, anxious or sad, remember menopausal symptoms are temporary. This mindset shift helps maintain equilibrium.

Developing practices that foster resilience before challenges occur eases adaptation when inevitable bumps in the road appear during menopause and midlife.

Positivity - Choosing Optimism

Deliberately focusing your mind on the positive counterbalances the tendency to fixate on negatives like menopausal symptoms, aging, or life stresses. Positivity boosts mood, relationships and health. Try:

Gratitude journaling - Jot down 3-5 things you're grateful for daily. Expressing gratitude, even for small joys, lifts depression, anxiety and stress.

Random acts of kindness - Doing good deeds boosts your own mood and wellbeing through the helper's high. Try volunteering.

Savor experiences - Deliberately pay close attention and appreciate pleasurable moments fully, engaging all your senses. Etch positive memories.

Limit media consumption - Reduce intake of negative news and limit social media use. These breed negativity bias and comparisons.

Watch your self-talk - Notice negative thought patterns and reframe them. Don't catastrophize or generalize. Dispute limiting beliefs.

Visualize your best self - Imagine how your best, most fulfilled self would think, feel and act, then work toward that ideal. Fake it until you make it!

Learn optimism strategies - Read books on positivity or take courses to learn how you generate explanatory styles. Reshape habitual thought patterns.

Practice affirmations - Post positive sayings and repeat uplifting mantras. Though cliché, they work by overriding ruminating thoughts.

Don't underestimate the power of deliberately cultivating positivity. It builds psychological strength to manage mood, motivation, relationships and overall wellbeing.

Self-Compassion - Being Kind to Yourself

Many women judge themselves harshly or feel guilty for declining energy, motivation, or ability during menopause. Practicing self-compassion provides emotional comfort. Self-compassion means:

- Giving yourself kindness, patience and understanding rather than being self-critical.

- Recognizing all people go through hard times and have flaws. You're not alone.

- Being mindfully present with discomfort versus overidentifying with negative thoughts about it. Acknowledge emotions without dramatizing.

Strategies to build self-compassion include:

Write a letter as if to a friend - Voice frustrations about menopausal challenges in a letter, then go back and rewrite it with loving understanding as if to a dear friend.

Talk to yourself compassionately - If you make a mistake or feel inadequate, notice harsh self-talk and consciously replace it with gentle, encouraging words as if consoling a friend.

Practice mindful self-soothing - When you feel bad, rub your arm, take deep breaths or meditate to calm and comfort yourself.

Develop self-care rituals- Do little acts like a candlelit bath or making a nurturing meal to care for yourself as you would someone you love.

Recognize shared humanity - When struggling, remind yourself "I am not alone, all humans suffer" to gain perspective.

Be your own best friend - Treat yourself as you would your closest confidant, with loyalty, cheerleading and kindness.

quiet inner critic and offer understanding. This emotional antidote relieves suffering.

Key Takeaways

- Foster resilience through community, self-care, optimism and meaning. This mental muscle helps you flexibly navigate challenges.

- Deliberately count blessings, perform acts of kindness, savor pleasures and limit media consumption to train your brain's positivity.

- Talk to yourself with compassion, understanding, and encouragement as you would a cherished friend to quiet harsh inner voices.

- Developing positivity, resilience and self-compassion provides the emotional strength to smooth menopause transitions.

In the next chapter, we'll explore practices for renewing relationships and connection with others during midlife changes. Our social connections provide crucial support.

Chapter 16: Strengthening Relationships

Our close relationships—with partners, children, friends and community—provide vital support as we navigate midlife changes. Investing in intimacy and social connections relieves stress and boosts resilience.

This chapter explores practices to proactively strengthen your relationships as roles evolve during menopause and midlife. Renewing bonds safeguards emotional health.

The Couple Connection

For partnered women, how your intimate relationship fares during menopause largely impacts your emotional experience. The quality of support and understanding your partner provides influences adjustment.

But you can also take steps to consciously build intimacy through:

Shared activities - Make regular time for novel, challenging experiences you both enjoy. Do a cooking class, hike, museum visit or weekend trip together. Novelty stimulates bonding hormones.

Express appreciation - Voicing genuine gratitude and praise for your partner's efforts renews fondness. Send a thank you text or leave love notes.

Physical touch - Non-sexual affection like hugging, hand-holding or cuddling maintains intimacy when sex wanes. Touch releases bonding oxytocin.

Thoughtful acts - Show love by cooking a favorite meal, running an errand, remembering an important date. Small gestures signal you hold your partner in mind.

Fun and laughter - Inject humor, playfulness and lighthearted moments to prevent negative drift. Laughter and goofiness release tension.

Shared goals - Have projects and passions you tackle as a team. Collaborating builds "we-ness" and accomplishment.

Open communication - Discuss feelings and experiences openly and often. Active listening and empathy prevents disconnect.

Compromise - Accept each person will change with aging. Negotiate conflicts fairly and seek win-win solutions.

Bond with others - Maintain outside friendships and interests so not everything relies solely on your partner. Mutual independence strengthens.

A proactive focus on intimacy skills prevents relationships from stagnating as life evolves. Seek counseling if needing help communicating or negotiating changes.

Strengthening Friendships

Having close, supportive friendships boosts mood and well-being during periods of stress. But neglecting friends while raising families or being absorbed in careers is common. Reinvesting in friends provides vital comfort.

Actions to take:

Reach out to old friends - Call, text or email old friends you've lost touch with. Plan reunions to reconnect. Share meaningful memories.

Make new friends - Changing life stages means making new friends with shared interests through classes, clubs, volunteering, or neighborhood groups.

Schedule regular activities - Plan regular walks, coffees, movie nights or other repeat activities so you stay connected consistently, not just sporadically.

Alternate hosting - Host friends at your home some nights, then enjoy nights hosted at theirs so obligations rotate. Potlucks split the work.

Remember important dates - Mark birthdays, family milestones, and important dates on your calendar. Reach out to support friends during hard times. Thoughtfulness matters.

Limit complaining - Venting feels relieving but constant complaining pushes people away. Balance troubles talk with positive subjects when together.

Follow through - If you commit to plans, even casually, honor them so friends feel valued, not blown off. Consistency builds trust.

Practice generosity - Be the friend who lends a listening ear, offers encouragement and provides help to others. Give the support you'd like.

Tending intentionally to friendships makes them an emotional refuge during tumultuous transitions like menopause. The sense of belonging benefits wellbeing.

Key Takeaways

- Proactively nurture your intimate relationship through shared activities, touch, laughter and communicating openly. Seek counseling if needed.

- Reaching out and dedicating time to friends, old and new, provides comfort and belonging during menopause.

- Tending to relationships helps maintain mental health and life satisfaction as roles evolve in midlife.

- The companionship of good friends and a supportive partner reduces stress and builds resilience to navigate changes.

In the next chapter, we'll explore reigniting your sensual side and sexuality after menopause so you can continue enjoying physical intimacy.

Chapter 17: Embracing Your Sexuality

Many women fear their sexuality will be diminished after menopause when fertility declines. But you can continue enjoying intimacy and passion by expanding definitions of sensuality, improving vaginal comfort, and communicating desires.

Let's explore strategies for embracing your sexuality fully throughout the menopausal transition and beyond.

Overcoming Vaginal Changes

Genitourinary symptoms like vaginal dryness, irritation, burning and pain with intercourse are common after menopause due to lower estrogen. But you have options to make intimacy comfortable:

Use lubricants - Apply water-based or silicone lubricants liberally to reduce friction that causes discomfort or pain. Avoid oils which degrade condoms. Reapply as needed.

Try vaginal moisturizers - These provide longer-lasting hydration and restore pH balance and elasticity when used regularly. Use up to twice weekly.

Discuss prescription estrogen - Local, low-dose vaginal estrogen reverses atrophy effectively for many women. Weigh hormone therapy risks and benefits.

Stay sexually active - Regular intercourse helps maintain elasticity of vaginal tissues. If penetrative sex is too painful, use dilators to stretch tissues.

Switch positions - Some positions, like woman on top, allow you to control depth of penetration. Go slowly. Switch when any activity becomes painful.

Communicate - Tell your partner when you experience pain so you can pause or try alternatives. Guide them on comfortable positions, pressure and techniques.

Don't silently endure penetrative sex if it hurts. Ongoing pain can cause vaginismus - involuntary tightening of pelvic floor muscles. Seek medical advice to address vulvovaginal discomfort.

Expanding Sensuality

Pleasure and intimacy need not revolve solely around penetrative sex. Broadening sensual horizons allows you to maintain fulfilling physical connection:

Prioritize foreplay - Savor sensual massage, kissing, manual and oral pleasuring. Don't rush into penetration before you feel fully aroused and your vagina is lubricated.

Try sensate focus exercises - Partners take turns giving sensual touch to different body parts without pressure for sexual response. This builds intimacy and arousal.

Experiment with sex toys - Vibrators, dildos, penis rings and massage toys add novelty and pleasure. Use lubricant to prevent friction.

Watch erotic videos together- Ethical feminist porn or curated collections celebrate female desire and body diversity. Viewing can help stimulate libido.

Incorporate role play- Take turns enacting fantasy scenarios to step out of everyday roles. Have fun taking on risqué personas or forbidden trysts.

Read or write erotica - Reading sexy stories activates imagination and fuels arousal. For inspiration, read anthologies by female authors or write your own.

Dance intimately - Slow dance, striptease and lap dances build sensual anticipation. Many couples find "vertical intercourse" satisfying.

Allowing intercourse to narrowly define sex sets up disappointment. Prioritize creative intimacy and whole-body sensuality instead.

Boosting Libido and Energy

If menopausal hormone changes or fatigue hinder your sex drive, natural remedies may help:

Exercise - Daily movement increases blood flow and energizes the body, often lifting libido. Strength training is ideal.

Manage stress - Unmanaged anxiety saps libido. Relaxation practices like meditation lower stress hormones that inhibit desire.

Get sufficient sleep - Being well-rested fuels the energy and motivation for sex. Prioritize 7-9 hours nightly.

Eat libido foods - Pomegranates, walnuts, oysters, dark chocolate, avocado, and watermelon contain compounds to boost circulation, endurance and arousal.

Try maca powder - This adaptogenic herb may help restore hormonal balance involved in regulating libido. Follow dosage guidelines.

Consider testosterone - If hormone testing reveals very low testosterone, supplementation under medical guidance may increase desire. Discuss carefully.

Use lubricants with stimulants - Products containing L-arginine help promote blood flow. Those with CBD provide anti-anxiety benefits.

Don't assume lackluster libido is inevitable. Troubleshoot contributing factors and incorporate natural pick-me-ups.

Key Takeaways

- Vaginal discomfort during sex due to menopausal changes can be managed with lubricants, local estrogen, staying active, and open communication.

- Expanding sensuality beyond intercourse to include oral sex, touching, sex toys and role play allows you to maintain intimacy when penetration is difficult.

- Stress management, proper sleep, exercise, supplements and recreational drugs can help reinvigorate libido if it declines.

- Prioritize pleasure, creativity and exploration to keep your sex life satisfying during menopause and beyond.

In the next chapter we'll explore practices for promoting purpose, growth and positive aging during midlife.

Chapter 18: Finding Meaning and Purpose

The midlife transition of menopause is an opportunity to evaluate your priorities and define the legacy you want to leave. Reflecting on how to infuse this stage with meaning allows you to move through it purposefully.

Let's explore practices for enriching this period of your life through service, creativity, wisdom development, and leaving a lasting contribution.

Making a Difference

Using your skills and experience to contribute to causes and people in need provides immense fulfillment after decades of investing in career and family. Ways to make a difference include:

Volunteer for a charity - Offer your time matching your passions, such as an animal shelter if you love animals. Micro-volunteering online is also easy and impactful.

Lend professional expertise - Consulting with nonprofits needing your career skills, such as marketing, technology or financial advice, leverages your knowledge.

Coach youth - Join organizations that pair adults with disadvantaged youth who benefit greatly from mentorship. Impart wisdom.

Assist the elderly - Volunteer with programs that help aging seniors with household tasks, social visits, or errands. Provide meaningful companionship.

Get politically active - Channel idealism into advocacy for issues you care about. Join activist groups and campaigns to create change.

Learn a support skill - Train to offer skills like psychotherapy, conflict mediation, or suicide prevention to serve your community. Many classes are free.

Beautify public spaces - Organize projects in your neighborhood to tag art, plant trees, collect litter or graffiti. Improving surroundings lifts spirits.

Teach or tutor - If you love learning and academia, teach community college courses, lead workshops or become a tutor to contribute your gifts.

Support family - Help overwhelmed siblings or grown children by babysitting, dogsitting, running errands, or providing respite care. Lend your calm.

Aligning life with purpose alleviates menopausal stresses and brings joy. Giving back also models good priorities for family.

Developing Wisdom

People associate wisdom with age through gained perspective and emotional intelligence. Actively cultivating wisdom helps you guide younger generations, achieving status as an honored elder. Elements include:

- Exceptional understanding of life gained via personal experiences

- Acknowledgement of uncertainty and limitations of knowledge

- Recognition of different contexts and viewpoints in decision-making

- Empathy, compassion and service to benefit the wellbeing of others

Ways to expand wisdom include:

Reflect on lessons learned - Review your life experiences to extract insights to guide future behavior and leadership.

Keep learning - Take educational courses and read widely to gain knowledge across disciplines. Mental stimulation strengthens cognitive abilities.

Observe thoughtfully - Notice other perspectives to see situations through different lenses. Withhold snap judgments.

Practice self-examination - Consider your biases, privilege, motivations and flaws through introspection. Know your shadows.

Develop emotional intelligence - Grow abilities like empathy, managing emotions, conflict resolution and listening. These are key in guidance roles.

Mentor others - The act of advising others based on your experience solidifies wisdom. Become a wise elder.

Spend time in nature - Observing natural patterns fosters systems thinking, humility and patience. Nature has much to teach us.

Wisdom develops through deliberate reflection, lifelong learning, emotional growth, patience with uncertainty, and serving as a guide.

Fostering Creativity and Play

Tapping into your creative side promotes joy, health, and brain stimulation to balance pragmatic midlife duties. Make time for:

Crafting - Find bliss in knitting, jewelry-making, macrame, calligraphy or other tactile crafts. Repetitive hands-on activities relax the mind.

Artistic hobbies - Take classes in pottery, painting, photography, sculpture or other arts you've always wanted to explore. Allow your playful side to emerge.

Home improvement projects - DIY skills not only upgrade your living space but provide a creative outlet. Build a garden bed, tile a backsplash, or paint an accent wall.

Writing - Try your hand at poetry, memoir, fiction or blogging to process emotions and distill wisdom from your experiences. Take a class to inspire you.

Dance - Joyful movement to music awakens your spirit and provides artistic release. Try line dancing, hip hop, tap, ballroom or free-form ecstatic dance.

Music - Play an instrument from your past, join a choir or drum circle, or learn something new like piano or ukulele. Making music engages the brain.

Acting or improv - Challenge yourself by taking an acting class or joining a local improv troupe. Theater builds confidence and self-expression.

Making creativity non-negotiable combats stress and provides pure enjoyment in the process of making art. What latent talents will you explore?

Key Takeaways

- Reflect on your legacy and how to leave the world and people better in this phase of influence. Volunteer for causes you care about.

- Actively cultivate wisdom through nature, observing different perspectives, emotional intelligence and lifelong learning.

- Tap into latent creative interests through arts, crafts, home projects, writing, music, dance and other right-brain activities.

- Infusing midlife with meaning, creativity and purpose ensures this transition enriches your life and legacy.

In the final chapter, we'll tie together all the elements needed to craft a balanced approach during menopause and beyond.

Part IV: Empowerment and Optimism

We've covered a lot of ground so far exploring the changes of menopause and proactive strategies to ease the transition across physical, mental, emotional and social realms. Now it's time to pull it all together.

This final section will provide a roadmap to integrate the diverse solutions into a tailored action plan optimized for your unique experience, symptoms and priorities.

You'll learn how to:

- Reframe mindsets and perspectives on menopause as a positive new beginning rather than an ending

- Shift focus from what is lost, like fertility and youth, to the many gains and freedoms of this life stage

- Build optimism and empowerment to take charge of your health during hormone changes

- Create a personalized plan of action targeting your top concerns and lifestyle goals

- Develop a holistic self-care regimen that nourishes your mind-body-spirit totality

- Embrace this transition as an opportunity for growth, self-discovery and living on your own terms

While menopause brings unavoidable changes, your power lies in how skillfully you adapt and leverage healthy solutions. With the right mindset and customized action plan, you can thrive through this passage.

When you reach the final pages, our hope is that you feel educated, uplifted and filled with a sense of possibility. Menopause signifies the start of a bold new chapter, not a farewell.

The tools are now in your hands - let's conclude by planning how to use them courageously!

Chapter 19: Reframing Perspective on Menopause

How you view menopause shapes your emotional experience of this transition. Seeing it as a loss or ending leaves you feeling discouraged. Reframing the narrative as an opportunity empowers you to shape this next chapter.

Let's explore how to shift perspective to one of optimism, growth, freedom and renewal. There are many gains to be realized!

From Loss to Potential

Menopause has historically been portrayed negatively, associated only with decline - the end of fertility, youth, attractiveness and femininity. But these limited portrayals no longer fit modern realities.

Today, empowered perspectives highlight the potential gains:

- Freedom from menstrual difficulties like cramps, PMS and heavy bleeding

- Liberation from worries about contraception and unplanned pregnancy

- Time and energy to refocus on your goals, talents and relationships

- Relief of symptoms if you had conditions like endometriosis that are estrogen-dependent

- Decreased risk for gynecological cancers fueled by hormones

- Emergence from child-rearing duties to pursue your own passions

- Flexibility for reinventing yourself and your path

- Opportunity to define yourself beyond motherhood or career labels

- Shift to a calmer pace if you choose, with less pressure

- Appreciation for aging and life phases that are temporary

- Development of wisdom and mastery over your life and mindset

Menopause signals entry into a phase of self-knowledge, authenticity, confidence and agency. It's a beginning, not an ending.

From "Surviving" to Thriving

Menopause has been portrayed as something to endure and survive, rather than truly master. But with the right strategies, you can move through it smoothly.

Rather than just coping, set intentions to:

- Emerge healthier, fitter, more energized than before

- Take time to nourish neglected parts of yourself

- Reset priorities to align values with actions

- Learn resilience and emotional agility skills

- Revel in freedom from past constraints

- Discover unexpected joys and talents

- Savor the reprieve from productivity pressures

- Deepen intimacy with self, partners and friends

- Infuse each day with creativity and passion

- Share your experiences to help other women

You have the power to not just survive, but thrive. Let go of rigid expectations and define success on your own terms. Allow some constructively messy reinvention!

From Anti-Aging to Pro-Aging

Looking through an anti-aging lens fuels fear and denial about natural aging. But you can shift to pro-aging - embracing increased wisdom, confidence and authenticity.

Adopt perspectives like:

- My value and worth is inherent, not dependent on youth.

- I aim to age skillfully with grace, wisdom and empowerment.

- I will challenge narrowly prescribed roles for "older" women.

- Each life stage has its unique gifts. None is better or worse.

- Aging allows me to live more fully aligned with my truth.

- I aim to master my health and wellbeing as I age.

- I will celebrate the added richness, depth and freedom that come with years of experience.

Aim not to look younger than your age, but to fully inhabit and optimize the age you are right now. Aging is a privilege some don't enjoy. Appreciate your lived years.

From Victim to Trailblazer

Finally, cast off outdated stereotypes of menopausal women as victims of raging hormones and ailing health. Instead, pioneer the trail for women to own this transition as a time of power, agency and wisdom.

Blaze new territories like:

- Challenging cultural myths about aging

- Advocating for women's health at midlife

- Forging your own ideas about meaning and fulfillment

- Exploring life's possibilities with childlike curiosity

- Learning new tools to care for your mind and body

- Being a mentor and wise elder for younger women

- Owning your seat at the table - you deserve to take up space!

- Making this passage easier for other women who follow

- Living as your truest, most actualized, authentic self

We stand at the dawn of a new era. How will you guide the way?

Key Takeaways

- Reframe menopause as a beginning, not an ending - one filled with freedoms, insights and new potential.

- Set your sights not just on surviving, but thriving through proactive self-care and lifestyle choices.

- Embrace aging as a privilege that allows you to live more fully aligned with your truth.

- Take up the mantle to challenge outdated myths and pioneer empowered perspectives on midlife.

As we conclude in our final chapter, the future is yours to shape with optimism and courage. Menopause marks the start of a bold new adventure unfold.

Chapter 20: Seeing Menopause as a New Beginning

You stand at the threshold of an exciting new chapter filled with possibility. Menopause heralds a rebirth - an opportunity to define life on your own terms, unencumbered by past constraints.

This transition can be your springboard to trying new things, focusing on your needs, and pursuing long-held dreams. Let's conclude by crafting an empowering action plan to launch your next adventure with vigor.

Reflecting on Your Goals

Begin by looking inward to re-evaluate priorities and intentions for this stage:

- What new interests do you wish to pursue?

- How do you want to grow and self-actualize?

- What relationships deserve more time and care?

- What parts of your life feel unbalanced or neglected?

- How do you wish to contribute your talents and wisdom?

- What legacy do you want to create or work unfinished?

- What makes your soul come alive and lights you up?

Envision how you want to feel - energized? Calm? Fulfilled? Then set goals to create those feelings. Dream big about how magnificent this chapter can become!

Crafting Your Action Plan

Now devise tactical steps to build the foundation for realizing your dreams and goals:

Sort top concerns - List your most bothersome menopausal symptoms. What physical or emotional issues most hinder wellbeing? Then rank which to tackle first.

Review solutions - Flip back through this book to compile remedies that address your priority issues. Note lifestyle changes, natural remedies, or medical options with proven benefits.

Schedule annual exam - Book a well-woman checkup to discuss symptoms and have hormone levels, nutrition, and disease risks assessed. Share the solutions you're most interested in.

Join support groups - Locate menopause education classes and support forums locally or online. Connecting with others provides solidarity plus ideas.

Identify resources - Search for providers covered by your insurance like therapists, nutritionists, trainers or specialists who can help build your action plan.

Address self-care gaps - Make time for neglected wellness basics like exercise, nutritious meals, restorative sleep, and stress management. Optimize foundations.

Hop on trends judiciously - Test new solutions like apps, wearables, telemedicine, or CBD with discretion. Find evidence-based options aligning with your healthcare philosophy.

Map milestones - Outline a realistic timeline for adopting changes in manageable increments. Prioritize steps with biggest impact. Periodically evaluate progress.

Optimizing Your Lifestyle

Beyond addressing symptoms, build regular habits and routines that nourish your mind, body and spirit to support the whole of your wellbeing:

Exercise often - Make daily movement non-negotiable - whether tennis, running, dancing, yoga or just walking outside. Pick activities bringing joy and community.

Eat nutritiously - Incorporate more plants, anti-inflammatory fats, gut-healthy fibers, and nutrient-dense foods into your diet. Hydrate well.

Get sufficient sleep - Prioritize 7-9 hours nightly, maintain sleep hygiene habits, and treat disorders contributing to fatigue. Nap if needed.

Stimulate your mind - Take classes, travel, learn new skills, read broadly, do puzzles. Mental stimulation strengthens cognition and builds neural pathways.

Practice mindfulness - Try meditation, breathwork, yoga, walking in nature. These practices reduce stress and cultivate serenity.

Do self-care rituals - Draw baths, massage sore muscles, light candles, listen to music - any acts nourishing your spirit.

Find your village - Surround yourself with supportive, positive friends and family who build you up and share your interests. Loneliness exacerbates malaise.

Volunteer or contribute - Offer your time and talent to meaningful causes. Doing good also delivers psychological benefits and purpose.

Have fun - Make play and laughter priorities. Try new adventures, games or hobbies that spark joy. Keep your inner child alive!

The path to an energized, purposeful and joy-filled midlife lies in diligently cultivating healthy routines and communities. Your action plan should holistically support your best life.

Key Takeaways

- Reflect first on your priorities, dreams and intentions for menopause and midlife. Envision your ideal state.

- Craft an action plan listing priority symptoms and solutions, assembling providers, joining groups, and outlining milestones.

- Complement your plan with lifestyle habits and relationships nurturing your physical, mental and spiritual health.

- Focus on infusing each day with positivity, vitality and meaning.

- You now have the knowledge and tools to skillfully chart your midlife journey. Bon voyage!

Conclusion: Entering Your Next Chapter with Confidence

When you began this book, you may have felt unsettled, hesitant or apprehensive about entering the uncharted waters of perimenopause and menopause.

Now armed with evidence-based information and proactive strategies, you can embark on this transition with knowledge, tools and confidence. While some degree of change is inevitable, you are no longer helpless.

We've covered the full landscape of what happens, what helps, and how to craft a tailored action plan. You have all the building blocks needed to navigate smoothly into your 40s, 50s and beyond.

Menopause is an opportunity to shed past constraints and rewrite the next chapters on your own terms. It's a threshold into a life stage with more freedom, wisdom and clarity about your true priorities.

Rather than something to survive, perimenopause and menopause signify a metamorphosis - emerging transformed, renewed and better aligned with your authentic self. Savor this period of increased agency over your life and wellbeing.

Midlife may bring role changes, but you have the chance to redefine those roles. Your identity need not be limited to career titles or parental duties. You are multidimensional. Clarify what matters, and have the courage to live it.

While some discomfort may accompany the hormonal transition, a balanced action plan mitigates the most bothersome symptoms. Some grit naturally comes with growth and change. But with the right mindset and solutions, you will gather your strength and thrive.

This book provided the blueprint - now the exciting work lies in putting solutions into practice. Lean on your community, care team and resources to bring your vision to life. You've got this!

We covered a lot of ground together, and I hope you feel equipped, uplifted and empowered. You stand at the entry to your next chapter, which extends long beyond menopause. How will you make it count? How will you live and age with grace, wisdom and vitality?

Your answers lie within. Heed your inner voice - it doesn't mislead. Keep your health and happiness paramount. The years ahead are filled with potential, purpose and possibility. Embrace this time of transformation with courage.

I wish you much joy, wisdom, empowerment and vitality as you chart this next phase of womanhood on your own terms. Your life's adventure continues!

Onward and upward always...

Resources

As you implement your menopause action plan, these resources offer helpful support. Tap into these organizations, services and materials to educate yourself further, connect with communities, and access providers.

Educational Organizations

North American Menopause Society (NAMS)

- Nonprofit focused on promoting women's health during midlife and beyond

- Publishes cutting-edge research on menopause and therapies

- Offers a clinician directory to find certified menopause practitioners

- Provides online education, newsletters, blogs and annual conference

www.menopause.org

The American College of Obstetricians and Gynecologists (ACOG)

- Professional association of OB/GYNs providing menopause education

- Offers content on menopause symptoms, risks, tests and treatment options

- Provides doctor-reviewed fact sheets and FAQs

- Helps locate ACOG member gynecologists

www.acog.org

Office on Women's Health (OWH), U.S. Department of Health and Human Services

- Leading federal agency providing menopause education and information

- Offers an e-newsletter, online content, webinars, and events

- Provides FAQs, consumer fact sheets, and health topic overviews on menopause

- Includes tips on choosing practitioners and tracking symptoms

www.womenshealth.gov/menopause

Support Organizations and Hotlines

Women's Health Initiative (WHI)

- Largest research study on health during and after menopause

- Offers information on participating in clinical trials

- Provides online courses, newsletters, and health risk assessment tools

1-800-411-8483

www.whi.org

National Osteoporosis Foundation

- Leading U.S. bone health and disease prevention foundation

- Provides online education, community forums and local support groups

- Offers information on prevention, treatment, diet and exercise for optimal bone health

1-800-231-4222

www.nof.org

Office on Women's Health Helpline

- Free, confidential helpline that provides menopause information

- Staffed by information specialists to answer women's health questions

- Service of the U.S. Department of Health and Human Services

1-800-994-9662

The North American Menopause Society Toll Free Call Center

- Provides science-based menopause health information

- Staffed by licensed healthcare providers and experts

- Can help you locate a certified menopause practitioner

1-800-774-5342

Online Communities and Chats

HealthBoards Menopause Community

- Online menopause forum with over 150,000 members

- Post questions, join discussions on symptoms, therapies

- Sections on sexuality, anxiety, relationships, etc.

www.healthboards.com/boards/menopause

Menopause Support Group on Daily Strength

- Supportive social network for women in perimenopause and menopause

- Share your story, connect with others worldwide going through the same issues

- Site offers various chronic health condition support groups

Mobile Apps

MenoPro

- Tracks period, symptoms, and lifestyle factors like mood, sex, and medications

- Analysis provides insights on how diet, exercise, etc. affect cycles

- Charts help identify perimenopause onset based on changing cycle length

My Menopause Doctor

- Tracks symptoms and generates custom reports to share with your doctor

- Assesses symptom severity using validated menopause rating scales

- Tracks hormone therapy if applicable

- Includes educational content

Menopause Coach

- Personalized 12-week program to relieve menopause symptoms naturally

- Incorporates diet, exercise, sleep, and stress management

- Provides access to menopause experts and community support

- Uses cognitive behavioral therapy techniques to change mindsets

Balance by Alloy

- All-encompassing women's health tracking app

- Logs cycles, symptoms, moods, sex, and medications
- Options for partner sharing and messaging
- Includes health courses and practitioner finder

Books

- Mayo Clinic The Menopause Solution by Dr. Jennifer Payne
- Menopocalypse by Amanda Thebe
- WomanCode by Alisa Vitti
- Estrogen Matters by Dr. Avrum Bluming
- The Wisdom of Menopause by Dr. Christiane Northrup
- Making Peace with Menopause by Susan Piver
- The Menopause Manifesto by Dr. Jen Gunter
- Menopause Confidential by Tara Allmen
- Your Best Age is Now by Dr. Robynne Chutkan

Podcasts

- The Menopause Whisperer
- Ready for the Change
- Mad About Menopause
- The Perimenopause Podcast
- Blazing & Aging
- Menopause & Me
- Menopause Barbie
- Making Menopause Easier

- My Menopause Journey

- The Midlife Muse

Wishing you health, empowerment and joy!

About the Author

Dr. Omolola Habib is a compassionate and knowledgeable naturopathic doctor who has made it her life's purpose to empower women to thrive during the menopause transition.

With an educational foundation spanning natural medicine, functional nutrition, and mindfulness-based wellness coaching, Dr. Habib takes a uniquely holistic approach to women's health. She recognizes that menopause affects the whole woman - body, mind and spirit - and customizes guidance to nurture each part.

Over her career, Dr. Habib has supported countless women in making smooth and graceful transitions into the next beautiful chapters of their lives. Her insights come not just from medical expertise, but from a place of deep empathy, intuition and care for the women she serves.

Her life's work is driven by a purpose close to her heart - empowering women through knowledge and sisterhood. She strives to lift outdated stigmas surrounding menopause and inspire women to own this transition courageously.

In "Navigating the Change," Dr. Habib distills decades of experience and wisdom into an accessible guide. With compassion and rigor, she equips readers to understand the changes ahead, implement customized solutions, and ultimately flourish through menopause.